"The Neem Nexus: Unveiling the Green Gold – From Tree to Oil"

"Harvesting Nature's Healing Power for Health and Sustainability"

BY

KATE MILES

INTRODUCTION

Overview of the Neem Plant:

The Neem tree, scientifically known as *Azadirachta indica*, is a versatile evergreen tree native to the Indian subcontinent. Revered for its multifaceted properties, the neem plant has earned the moniker "Nature's Pharmacy" due to its extensive uses in traditional medicine, agriculture, and various industries.

Botanical Characteristics:

Taxonomy: Belonging to the *Meliaceae* family, the neem tree shares botanical ties with mahogany.

Morphology: Neem trees typically reach heights of 15 to 20 meters, boasting a dense crown of pinnate leaves and fragrant white flowers.

Geographical Distribution:

Neem thrives in tropical and subtropical regions, finding a natural habitat in countries like India, Bangladesh, Sri Lanka, and parts of Africa.

Traditional and Cultural Significance:

Ayurvedic Tradition: Neem occupies a revered place in Ayurveda, the ancient Indian system of medicine, where various parts of the plant are used for their therapeutic properties.

Rituals and Symbolism: In some cultures, neem is associated with purification rituals and considered a symbol of health and well-being.

Ecological Impact:

Biodiversity Support: Neem contributes to biodiversity by providing habitat and sustenance for various organisms.

Soil Improvement: The fallen neem leaves act as a natural fertilizer, enhancing soil fertility.

Pest-Repellent Properties:

Neem is renowned for its natural pest-repellent qualities, acting as a deterrent against a range of insects. This has led to its extensive use in organic and sustainable agriculture.

Medicinal Properties:

Antimicrobial: Neem exhibits antimicrobial properties, making it a key ingredient in traditional remedies for skin ailments and infections.

Anti-inflammatory: Compounds in neem have anti-inflammatory effects, contributing to its use in addressing various health conditions.

Understanding the comprehensive nature of the neem plant is essential for unlocking its potential across diverse fields, from traditional medicine to sustainable agriculture and beyond.

Historical Significance of the Neem Plant:

The historical roots of the neem plant stretch deep into the cultural and medicinal tapestry of ancient civilizations, particularly in the Indian subcontinent. Revered for its multifaceted benefits, neem has played a crucial role in various aspects of human life throughout the ages.

Ayurvedic Heritage:

Neem holds a prominent place in Ayurveda, the ancient Indian system of medicine, where it is referred to as "Sarva Roga Nivarini" – the universal healer of ailments. Ayurvedic texts, dating back thousands of years, document the therapeutic properties of neem in treating a myriad of health conditions.

Traditional Medicine:

Across India and neighboring regions, communities have incorporated neem into traditional medicine for centuries. Its leaves, bark, seeds, and oil have been used to create remedies for skin disorders, fevers, digestive issues, and more.

Agricultural Practices:

Neem's significance extends to agriculture, where its pest-repelling properties have been harnessed for generations. Farmers have employed neem-based formulations to protect crops and enhance soil fertility.

Religious and Cultural Symbolism:

In Hinduism, the neem tree is often associated with various deities and considered sacred. It is not uncommon to find neem trees in temple courtyards, emphasizing their spiritual importance.

Historical Texts and References:

Ancient Indian texts such as the Vedas and Puranas contain references to neem, showcasing its presence in the daily lives of people across millennia. These texts often highlight neem's purifying and health-promoting qualities.

Global Spread:

As trade routes expanded, so did the recognition of neem beyond its place of origin. The tree's reputation for medicinal and agricultural benefits contributed to its adoption in various cultures across Asia, Africa, and the Middle East.

Modern Scientific Validation:

In more recent times, scientific research has validated many of the historical claims regarding neem's medicinal and agricultural efficacy. This has led to a renewed interest in harnessing neem's potential for sustainable practices and healthcare.

The historical significance of the neem plant underscores its enduring role in human civilization, from ancient healing traditions to contemporary applications in agriculture and beyond.

Table of Contents

CHAPTER 1

BOTANICAL INSIGHTS

Taxonomy and Classification of the Neem Plant (*Azadirachta indica*):

The neem plant, scientifically known as *Azadirachta indica*, belongs to the Meliaceae family. Taxonomy involves the classification of living organisms based on shared characteristics, and the neem tree fits into a specific hierarchy within this system.

Kingdom: Plantae

Neem, like all plants, falls under the Kingdom Plantae, which encompasses a diverse array of multicellular, eukaryotic organisms capable of photosynthesis.

Division: Magnoliophyta (Angiosperms)

Angiosperms are flowering plants, and neem is classified within this division. These plants produce seeds enclosed within a protective ovary, often housed in a flower.

Class: Magnoliopsida (Dicotyledons)

Dicotyledons, or dicots, represent a class of angiosperms characterized by having two cotyledons (seed leaves) in their embryos. Neem is a dicotyledonous plant.

Order: Sapindales

Neem belongs to the order Sapindales, a diverse group of flowering plants that includes species like mangoes and cashews. The order is known for its economic and ecological importance.

Family: Meliaceae

Within the order Sapindales, neem is a member of the Meliaceae family. This family is commonly referred to as the mahogany family, and it includes other economically valuable trees.

Genus: Azadirachta

The genus Azadirachta encompasses various species, but Azadirachta indica is the specific species associated with the neem tree. This genus is known for its medicinal and pesticidal properties.

Species: *Azadirachta indica*

Azadirachta indica is the species name that specifically identifies the neem tree. It is under this species that the unique characteristics and attributes of the neem plant are classified.

Understanding the taxonomy and classification of the neem plant provides insights into its evolutionary relationships with other organisms and its place within the plant kingdom. This classification system helps botanists, researchers, and enthusiasts categorize and study the diversity of life on Earth.

Morphology of the Neem Plant (*Azadirachta indica*): The morphology of the neem plant, *Azadirachta indica*, encompasses a distinctive set of features that contribute to its recognition and functionality. From its leaves to its flowers and seeds, each part plays a crucial role in the ecological and practical significance of the neem tree.

Leaves:

Neem leaves are pinnately compound, meaning they are arranged in pairs along the stem, with each pair comprising multiple leaflets. The leaflets are lance-shaped with serrated edges, and they give the tree a feathery appearance.

Bark:

The bark of the neem tree is brown to grayish-brown and possesses a rough texture. It can be deeply furrowed, providing protection to the inner layers of the tree.

Flowers:

Neem flowers are small, white, and fragrant. They are arranged in clusters, forming delicate inflorescences. The blossoms are often conspicuous against the backdrop of the tree's dense foliage.

Fruits:

Neem produces drupe-like fruits that are oval or elongated. These fruits contain a single seed and have a greenish-yellow hue when young, maturing to a yellowish-brown color.

Seeds:

Neem seeds are the source of neem oil. They are enclosed within the fleshy fruit and have a kernel covered by a thin seed coat. The seeds are rich in oil, which is extracted for various purposes.

Growth Form:

Neem trees typically have a straight and tall trunk with a spreading crown. The canopy is dense and provides ample shade. The overall growth form of the neem tree is well-adapted to thrive in tropical and subtropical climates.

Roots:

Neem trees have a deep and extensive root system, allowing them to access water from lower soil layers. The roots also play a role in stabilizing the tree.

Understanding the morphology of the neem plant is essential for recognizing it in its natural habitat and for harnessing its various benefits. Whether it's the distinctive compound leaves, fragrant flowers, or oil-rich seeds, each morphological feature contributes to the ecological and practical importance of the neem tree.

CHAPTER 2
NEEM'S ECOLOGICAL IMPACT

Environmental Benefits of the Neem Plant (*Azadirachta indica*):

The neem plant, *Azadirachta indica*, offers a range of environmental benefits, making it a valuable asset in promoting ecological balance and sustainable practices. Here are some key environmental advantages associated with the neem tree:

Biodiversity Support:

Neem trees provide a habitat for various organisms, including birds, insects, and microorganisms. This biodiversity support contributes to the overall health and resilience of ecosystems.

Soil Improvement:

The fallen leaves of the neem tree act as a natural fertilizer, enriching the soil with organic matter. This organic input enhances soil fertility and promotes healthy microbial activity in the rhizosphere.

Erosion Control:

The extensive root system of neem trees helps bind the soil, preventing erosion. This is particularly beneficial in regions prone to soil degradation and loss.

Carbon Sequestration:

Like all trees, neem contributes to carbon sequestration by absorbing carbon dioxide during photosynthesis. This helps mitigate the impacts of climate change by reducing the concentration of greenhouse gases in the atmosphere.

Natural Pest Control:

Neem possesses natural pesticidal properties, acting as a deterrent against a wide range of pests. This reduces the reliance on synthetic pesticides, which can have detrimental effects on the environment and non-target species.

Water Conservation:

The deep root system of neem enables it to access water from lower soil layers. This can be beneficial in water-stressed regions, contributing to water conservation efforts.

Agroforestry Practices:

Neem is often integrated into agroforestry systems, where it serves multiple purposes such as providing shade, improving soil fertility, and acting as a windbreak. This promotes sustainable land use practices.

Medicinal Plant Diversity:

The medicinal properties of neem contribute to the diversity of plant-based remedies in traditional and modern medicine. Preserving such biodiversity is essential for the discovery of new pharmaceutical compounds.

Low Environmental Impact:

Neem-based products, including pesticides and fertilizers, are known for their biodegradability and low environmental impact. This contrasts with some synthetic alternatives that can have long-lasting and harmful effects.

By virtue of its ecological contributions, the neem plant exemplifies the concept of sustainable coexistence, offering a range of environmental benefits that extend beyond its individual presence.

Neem in Agroecology: Harnessing Nature's Wisdom for Sustainable Agriculture

Agroecology, the practice of applying ecological principles to agricultural systems, finds a powerful ally in the neem tree (*Azadirachta indica*). Neem's multifaceted properties contribute significantly to sustainable farming practices, promoting environmental health and the well-being of crops. Here's a closer look at how neem is integrated into agroecological systems:

Natural Pest Control:

Neem is renowned for its insect-repelling properties. Neem-based pesticides act as a natural deterrent against a wide range of pests, helping farmers reduce reliance on synthetic chemical pesticides. This not only protects crops but also minimizes the environmental impact associated with conventional pest control methods.

Soil Enhancement:

Neem leaves are a rich source of organic matter, and when used as a mulch, they contribute to soil fertility. The gradual decomposition of neem leaves releases nutrients into the soil, enhancing its structure and promoting microbial activity. This, in turn, improves water retention and nutrient availability for plants.

Nitrogen Fixation:

Neem trees have the ability to fix atmospheric nitrogen, a vital nutrient for plant growth. Planting neem in agroecosystems can support nitrogen cycling, enriching the soil with this essential element and promoting healthier plant development.

Agroforestry Systems:

Integrating neem into agroforestry systems provides additional benefits. Neem's canopy provides shade, reducing temperature stress on crops. The deep root system helps prevent soil erosion, and the fallen leaves act as a natural fertilizer, creating a more sustainable and resilient farming environment.

Companion Planting:

Neem's pest-repelling properties extend to companion planting strategies. By strategically planting neem trees or incorporating neem extracts into the planting scheme, farmers can create a protective environment that discourages pests and supports the overall health of the agroecosystem.

Sustainable Crop Management:

The use of neem-based formulations for crop protection aligns with the principles of integrated pest management (IPM). This holistic approach emphasizes the importance of ecological balance and reduces the negative impacts of pest control on non-target organisms.

Disease Resistance:

Neem has demonstrated antifungal and antibacterial properties. When applied preventively, neem formulations can contribute to disease resistance in crops, reducing the need for chemical fungicides and antibiotics.

Incorporating neem into agroecological practices not only aligns with sustainable farming principles but also highlights the potential for nature-inspired solutions in agriculture. By tapping into the ecological benefits of the neem tree, agroecology embraces a holistic approach that harmonizes with natural processes for long-term agricultural sustainability.

CHAPTER 3
NUTRITIONAL AND MEDICINAL PROPERTIES

Neem's Nutritional Value: Exploring the Healthful Components of *Azadirachta indica*

While primarily renowned for its medicinal and pesticidal properties, the neem plant (*Azadirachta indica*) also possesses nutritional value, offering a range of beneficial compounds. Though not a traditional food source, various parts of the neem tree have been used in traditional medicine to provide health benefits. Here's an overview of neem's nutritional components:

Neem Leaves:

Antioxidants: Neem leaves contain antioxidants, including flavonoids and polyphenols, which help combat oxidative stress in the body.

Vitamins: Neem leaves are a source of vitamin C, supporting immune function, and vitamin A, important for vision and skin health.

Neem Seeds:

Fatty Acids: Neem seeds are rich in fatty acids, including oleic acid, linoleic acid, and palmitic acid. These contribute to overall health and are essential for various bodily functions.

Proteins: Neem seeds contain proteins, providing amino acids necessary for the body's growth and repair processes.

Neem Oil:

Essential Fatty Acids: Neem oil is particularly high in essential fatty acids, such as omega-6 and omega-9, which are beneficial for skin health.

Vitamin E: Neem oil contains vitamin E, known for its antioxidant properties and its role in promoting skin health.

Neem Flowers:

Nutrient Content: Neem flowers contain various nutrients, adding to the overall nutritional profile of the plant. They are often used in traditional medicine for their health-promoting properties.

Neem Bark:

Bioactive Compounds: Neem bark contains compounds like tannins and alkaloids, contributing to its medicinal properties. While not a primary source of nutrition, these bioactive compounds play a role in traditional remedies.

Traditional Uses:

Across cultures, neem leaves have been traditionally consumed in various forms, such as neem tea or extracts. These preparations are valued for their potential health benefits and are sometimes incorporated into wellness practices.

While not a staple in the human diet, the nutritional components found in different parts of the neem tree contribute to its holistic value. As research continues, the exploration of neem's nutritional properties may uncover additional health benefits and applications beyond its well-established roles in traditional medicine and agriculture.

Medicinal Uses and Traditional Practices of the Neem Plant (*Azadirachta indica*):

The neem plant, revered as a "pharmacy tree" in traditional medicine, has a rich history of therapeutic applications in various cultures. Its diverse range of bioactive compounds contributes to its effectiveness in addressing an array of health concerns. Here are some key medicinal uses and traditional practices associated with the neem plant:

Skin Conditions:

Anti-Inflammatory Properties: Neem is employed in treating skin conditions like eczema, psoriasis, and acne due to its potent anti-inflammatory properties. Neem oil and neem leaf extracts are applied topically to alleviate redness and irritation.

Antimicrobial Agent:

Antibacterial and Antifungal Properties: Neem is recognized for its ability to combat bacterial and fungal infections. Traditional practices involve using neem-based preparations for wounds, cuts, and skin infections.

Oral Health:

Dental Care: Neem's antibacterial properties extend to oral health. Chewing neem twigs or using neem-based toothpaste is a traditional practice for promoting gum health, reducing plaque, and preventing cavities.

Immune Support:

Immunomodulatory Effects: Neem is believed to support the immune system. Traditional remedies include neem supplements or infusions during times of illness to aid in recovery.

Fever and Malaria:

Antipyretic Properties: Neem has been traditionally used to reduce fever. Neem leaves or neem-based formulations are often administered to individuals with febrile conditions.

Digestive Health:

Antiparasitic Effects: Neem is valued for its antiparasitic properties, and traditional practices involve using neem to address gastrointestinal issues caused by parasites. Neem extracts are believed to have a cleansing effect on the digestive tract.

Diabetes Management:

Blood Sugar Regulation: Neem is explored for its potential in diabetes management. Traditional remedies involve the use of neem leaves or neem supplements to help regulate blood sugar levels.

Reproductive Health:

Contraceptive Properties: In some traditional systems, neem has been explored for its contraceptive properties. Neem oil and neem extracts are used in various formulations.

Anti-Inflammatory and Analgesic Uses:

Pain Relief: Neem has analgesic properties and is traditionally used to alleviate pain. This includes conditions such as arthritis and muscle aches.

Ayurvedic Formulations:

Neem is a key ingredient in numerous Ayurvedic formulations. Traditional Ayurvedic practitioners utilize neem in various preparations, including decoctions, powders, and oils, tailored to specific health needs.

While neem's traditional uses are deeply rooted in cultural practices, ongoing scientific research continues to explore and validate its medicinal properties, shedding light on the potential integration of neem-based remedies into modern healthcare practices.

CHAPTER 4

NEEM OIL EXTRACTION PROCESS

Harvesting Neem Seeds: Nurturing the Source of Nature's Green Gold

Harvesting neem seeds is a crucial step in unlocking the valuable resource known as neem oil, celebrated for its diverse applications in agriculture, health, and beauty. Here's a closer look at the process of harvesting neem seeds:

Maturity of the Neem Tree:

Neem trees typically start bearing fruits around 3 to 5 years of age, although full maturity may take longer. Harvesting is most productive when the tree is mature and actively producing seeds.

Identification of Mature Seeds:

Mature neem seeds are found within the fleshy drupe-like fruits produced by the neem tree. The fruits are typically yellowish or greenish when young, gradually turning a yellow-brown color as they mature. Ripe fruits are plump and emit a distinct, pungent aroma.

Collection of Fallen Fruits:

Neem fruits often fall from the tree when they are ripe. Harvesters can collect these fallen fruits from the ground. Care should be taken to gather fruits that are free from damage or rot.

Manual Harvesting:

In some cases, especially for small-scale operations, neem fruits may be manually harvested directly from the tree. This requires careful handling to avoid damage to the seeds.

Extraction of Seeds from the Fruit:

Neem seeds are extracted from the fruit pulp, which can be done manually or through mechanical means. Once removed, the seeds are thoroughly cleaned to eliminate any remaining pulp.

Drying the Seeds:

After extraction, neem seeds are spread out in a well-ventilated area to dry. Proper drying is essential to reduce moisture content and prevent mold formation. Sun drying is a common method, but care should be taken to avoid excessive heat, which could compromise the quality of the oil.

Storage of Neem Seeds:

Dried neem seeds are stored in cool, dry conditions to maintain their quality. Proper storage helps prevent mold growth and preserves the viability of the seeds for future processing.

Oil Extraction:

Neem seeds are the primary source of neem oil. The oil extraction process involves crushing or pressing the seeds to release the oil. Cold-pressing methods are often preferred to preserve the oil's nutritional and medicinal properties.

By-Products Utilization:

Neem seed cake, a by-product of oil extraction, is rich in nutrients and can be used as organic fertilizer. This sustainable practice ensures minimal waste in the neem oil production process.

Harvesting neem seeds is a meticulous process that requires careful attention to timing and handling. This sustainable approach not only yields valuable neem oil but also allows for the utilization of by-products, contributing to a more holistic and eco-friendly production cycle.

Neem Oil Extraction Techniques: Tapping into Nature's Green Gold

Neem oil, often referred to as "Nature's Pharmacy in a Bottle," is extracted from the seeds of the neem tree (*Azadirachta indica*). The oil extraction process involves various techniques, each designed to preserve the integrity of the oil and its beneficial properties. Here's an exploration of common neem oil extraction methods:

Cold-Pressing:

Process: Cold-pressing is a traditional and widely used method for neem oil extraction. It involves mechanically pressing the neem seeds at low temperatures, typically below 122°F (50°C).

Advantages: This method retains the oil's natural color, odor, and bioactive compounds, ensuring a high-quality end product with optimal therapeutic benefits.

Applications: Cold-pressed neem oil is favored in cosmetic and medicinal applications due to its purity and preservation of bioactive compounds.

Solvent Extraction:

Process: Solvent extraction involves using chemical solvents, such as hexane, to dissolve the oil from the neem seeds. The solvent is then evaporated to leave behind the neem oil.

Advantages: This method is efficient and yields a higher quantity of oil compared to cold-pressing.

Considerations: The use of chemical solvents raises concerns about residues in the final product, and steps must be taken to ensure thorough solvent removal.

Steam Distillation:

Process: In steam distillation, steam is passed through the crushed neem seeds, vaporizing the essential oil components. The steam is then condensed to collect the neem oil.

Advantages: This method is commonly used for extracting essential oils and can preserve some of the aromatic compounds found in neem oil.

Limitations: Steam distillation may not extract the full spectrum of bioactive compounds present in neem oil.

Supercritical Fluid Extraction (SFE):

Process: Supercritical fluid extraction involves using supercritical carbon dioxide to extract neem oil from the seeds. Under specific temperature and pressure conditions, carbon dioxide behaves as both a liquid and a gas, allowing efficient extraction.

Advantages: SFE is a precise and environmentally friendly method that produces high-quality neem oil with minimal solvent residues.

Considerations: The equipment for SFE can be expensive, making this method less accessible for small-scale operations.

Mechanical Expeller Press:

Process: Similar to cold-pressing, mechanical expeller presses crush neem seeds to extract the oil. However, expeller pressing often involves higher temperatures.

Advantages: It's a cost-effective method suitable for larger-scale operations.

Considerations: The higher temperatures used in some expeller pressing methods may affect the preservation of certain bioactive compounds.

Selecting the appropriate neem oil extraction method depends on factors such as the desired end product, scale of production, and consideration of environmental and quality standards. Whether through traditional cold-pressing or modern supercritical fluid extraction, each method plays a role in bringing forth the diverse benefits of neem oil.

CHAPTER 5
CHEMICAL COMPOSITION OF NEEM OIL

Active Compounds in Neem: Unlocking the Therapeutic Arsenal of *Azadirachta indica*

The neem plant (*Azadirachta indica*) is a treasure trove of bioactive compounds, each contributing to its renowned medicinal and pesticidal properties. These active compounds, found in various parts of the neem tree, collectively create a potent therapeutic arsenal. Here's an exploration of some key active compounds in neem:

Azadirachtin:

Function: Azadirachtin is the most well-known and researched compound in neem. It acts as a potent insect repellent and disruptor of insect feeding and molting.

Applications: Widely used in organic farming, azadirachtin is a key component of neem-based pesticides.

Nimbin:

Function: Nimbin possesses anti-inflammatory and analgesic properties, making it valuable for addressing various inflammatory conditions.

Applications: Traditional medicine utilizes nimbin for pain relief and as an anti-inflammatory agent.

Nimbidin:

Function: Nimbidin exhibits antipyretic (fever-reducing) and anti-inflammatory effects. It also contributes to neem's antibacterial properties.

Applications: Used traditionally for fever reduction and in skin care for its anti-inflammatory benefits.

Quercetin:

Function: Quercetin is a flavonoid with antioxidant properties, helping to neutralize free radicals in the body.

Applications: Its antioxidant nature contributes to neem's overall health-promoting effects.

Beta-Sitosterol:

Function: Beta-sitosterol has anti-inflammatory properties and is known to support prostate health.

Applications: Found in neem seeds, beta-sitosterol contributes to the overall health benefits of neem oil.

Salannin:

Function: Salannin acts as an insect feeding deterrent and contributes to neem's insecticidal properties.

Applications: Supports neem's role in pest control and agriculture.

Polysaccharides:

Function: Polysaccharides contribute to neem's immunomodulatory effects, supporting the immune system.

Applications: Traditional medicine utilizes neem for immune support and overall health.

Gedunin:

Function: Gedunin has antimalarial properties and contributes to neem's ability to combat certain parasites.

Applications: Traditional remedies may involve neem for its antiparasitic effects.

Azadirone:

Function: Azadirone exhibits antifungal properties, contributing to neem's effectiveness against certain fungi.

Applications: Used in traditional medicine for fungal infections and skin conditions.

Triterpenoids:

Function: Triterpenoids, including limonoids, contribute to neem's antiviral and anticancer properties.

Applications: Research is ongoing to explore the potential therapeutic applications of neem triterpenoids.

The synergy of these active compounds makes neem a versatile botanical remedy. Whether used in traditional medicine, agriculture, or skincare, neem's diverse bioactive profile continues to inspire research and harness its potential for human and environmental well-being.

Pharmacological Properties of Neem (*Azadirachta indica*): A Holistic Healing Hub

The pharmacological properties of neem extend far beyond its traditional uses, embracing a broad spectrum of therapeutic effects that have captured the attention of modern research. Here's an exploration of the pharmacological properties that make neem a holistic healing hub:

Antimicrobial Activity:

Overview: Neem demonstrates potent antimicrobial properties against bacteria, viruses, and fungi.

Mechanism: Compounds like azadirachtin, nimbin, and nimbidin contribute to inhibiting the growth and reproduction of various microbes.

Applications: Neem is used in traditional medicine for treating bacterial and fungal infections. Modern research explores its potential in developing new antimicrobial agents.

Anti-Inflammatory Effects:

Overview: Neem exhibits anti-inflammatory properties, contributing to its efficacy in addressing inflammatory conditions.

Mechanism: Nimbidin and other compounds in neem help modulate inflammatory pathways and reduce inflammation.

Applications: Used traditionally for conditions involving inflammation, modern studies explore neem's potential in managing inflammatory disorders.

Antioxidant Capacity:

Overview: Neem is rich in antioxidants that help neutralize free radicals in the body.

Mechanism: Compounds like quercetin and beta-sitosterol contribute to neem's antioxidant activity.

Applications: The antioxidant nature of neem supports overall health and may play a role in preventing oxidative stress-related diseases.

Immunomodulatory Effects:

Overview: Neem has immunomodulatory properties, influencing the activity of the immune system.

Mechanism: Polysaccharides in neem contribute to the modulation of immune responses.

Applications: Traditional medicine utilizes neem for immune support, and ongoing research explores its potential in immunotherapy.

Antiviral Properties:

Overview: Neem shows antiviral activity against various viruses.

Mechanism: Compounds like triterpenoids contribute to inhibiting viral replication.

Applications: Neem is explored for its potential in antiviral therapies and as a preventive measure against certain viral infections.

Antidiabetic Effects:

Overview: Neem exhibits potential in managing diabetes.

Mechanism: Compounds in neem may help regulate blood sugar levels.

Applications: Traditional remedies involve neem for diabetes management, and ongoing research explores its role in supporting conventional diabetes treatments.

Anticancer Properties:

Overview: Neem compounds, including triterpenoids, show promise in inhibiting cancer cell growth.

Mechanism: Triterpenoids contribute to inducing apoptosis (programmed cell death) in cancer cells.

Applications: Neem is under investigation for its potential as an adjuvant therapy in cancer treatment.

Antiparasitic Effects:

Overview: Neem demonstrates efficacy against various parasites.

Mechanism: Gedunin and other compounds contribute to neem's antiparasitic activity.

Applications: Used traditionally for parasitic infections, neem is explored for its role in developing antiparasitic medications.

As research advances, the pharmacological properties of neem continue to unveil new possibilities in healthcare and wellness. The holistic nature of neem's healing potential positions it as a valuable resource in the quest for natural and sustainable therapeutic solutions.

CHAPTER 6

APPLICATIONS OF NEEM OIL

Neem in Agriculture and Pest Control: Cultivating Sustainability

Neem (*Azadirachta indica*) stands as a green guardian in agriculture, offering a natural and sustainable approach to pest control and soil enhancement. Its diverse array of bioactive compounds makes it a valuable asset for promoting healthy crops and minimizing the impact of pests. Here's an exploration of neem's role in agriculture and pest control:

Pest Repellent Properties:

Azadirachtin's Impact: Azadirachtin, a key compound in neem, disrupts the feeding and reproductive patterns of insects, acting as a potent natural insect repellent.

Broad Spectrum: Neem's pesticidal properties extend to a wide range of pests, including aphids, caterpillars, mites, and beetles.

Biopesticide Formulations:

Neem Oil Sprays: Neem oil, extracted from neem seeds, is a versatile biopesticide. Diluted neem oil can be sprayed on crops to control pests without harming beneficial insects.

Seed Coating: Treating seeds with neem formulations protects them from soil-dwelling pests during germination.

Nematode Control:

Nimbin's Role: Nimbin, another bioactive compound in neem, contributes to its effectiveness against nematodes.

Soil Amendment: Incorporating neem cake (residue after oil extraction) into the soil helps manage nematode populations and improves soil fertility.

Fungicidal Properties:

Azadirachtin's Antifungal Action: Neem's antifungal properties, attributed to compounds like azadirachtin, make it effective against various plant pathogens.

Preventing Crop Diseases: Neem-based formulations are used to prevent and manage fungal diseases, such as powdery mildew and rust.

Soil Enhancement:

Organic Fertilizer: Neem cake, a by-product of neem oil extraction, serves as an excellent organic fertilizer. It enriches the soil with essential nutrients and improves its structure.

Microbial Activity: Neem cake promotes beneficial microbial activity in the soil, contributing to overall soil health.

Sustainable Agricultural Practices:

Reduced Chemical Dependency: Neem's role in pest control allows for a reduction in the use of synthetic pesticides, promoting environmentally friendly and sustainable agricultural practices.

Integrated Pest Management (IPM): Neem fits well into IPM strategies, emphasizing the use of multiple pest control methods for a balanced and sustainable approach.

Agroforestry and Windbreaks:

Shade and Wind Protection: Neem trees, when strategically planted in agroforestry systems, provide shade and act as windbreaks. This helps create a microclimate conducive to crop growth.

Diversification: Integrating neem into agroforestry systems enhances biodiversity and supports sustainable land use.

Resistance Management:

Reducing Pesticide Resistance: Neem's multiple modes of action against pests make it a valuable tool in resistance management, helping to combat the development of resistance to chemical pesticides.

Neem's multifaceted contributions to agriculture go beyond pest control; it fosters a holistic and sustainable approach that aligns with the principles of ecological balance and long-term soil fertility. As a green ally in the field, neem continues to play a pivotal role in cultivating a sustainable and resilient agricultural landscape.

Neem in Health and Beauty Products: Unveiling Nature's Wellness Elixir

Neem (*Azadirachta indica*) transcends its traditional roots to become a key ingredient in a variety of health and beauty products. Revered for its therapeutic properties, neem contributes to formulations that cater to skincare, haircare, and overall well-being. Here's an exploration of neem's presence in health and beauty products:

Skincare Products:

Neem Oil in Lotions and Creams: Neem oil, rich in essential fatty acids and antioxidants, is a common ingredient in lotions and creams. It helps moisturize the skin and provides nourishment.

Anti-Acne Face Washes: Neem's antimicrobial properties make it a popular choice in face washes designed to combat acne and promote clear skin.

Haircare Formulations:

Neem Oil in Shampoos: Neem oil's antibacterial and antifungal properties make it beneficial in shampoos, addressing scalp issues like dandruff and promoting a healthy scalp.

Conditioners and Hair Masks: Neem extracts are often incorporated into conditioners and hair masks for their moisturizing and nourishing effects on hair.

Anti-Aging Creams:

Antioxidant-Rich Formulas: Neem's antioxidant compounds, including quercetin and beta-sitosterol, contribute to anti-aging creams. They help combat free radicals, reducing the signs of aging.

Toothpaste and Oral Care:

Neem in Toothpaste: Neem's antibacterial properties make it a suitable ingredient in toothpaste, promoting oral hygiene and preventing dental issues.

Mouthwashes and Oral Rinses: Neem extracts are utilized in oral care products for their ability to combat bacteria and support gum health.

Medicinal Balms and Ointments:

Topical Healing: Neem is incorporated into balms and ointments for its anti-inflammatory and antimicrobial properties, making it effective for soothing skin irritations, cuts, and insect bites.

Eczema and Psoriasis Creams: Neem's skin-calming properties are harnessed in creams designed to alleviate symptoms of conditions like eczema and psoriasis.

Neem Soap:

Antibacterial Cleansing: Neem soap is popular for its antibacterial properties, offering a natural alternative for cleansing and maintaining skin health.

Acne Control: The antimicrobial effects of neem make it an ideal choice for soaps targeting acne-prone skin.

Ayurvedic Formulations:

Traditional Wellness Products: Neem is a staple in Ayurvedic formulations, contributing to herbal remedies and wellness products that support overall health.

Herbal Supplements: Neem supplements, often in the form of capsules or powders, are utilized for their potential immune-boosting and detoxifying effects.

Natural Insect Repellents:

Neem-Based Repellent Sprays: Neem's insect-repelling properties extend to health and beauty products such as natural insect repellent sprays, offering protection against mosquitoes and other pests.

As consumers increasingly seek natural and sustainable options, neem's presence in health and beauty products continues to grow. Its versatility, combined with a rich array of beneficial compounds, positions neem as a sought-after ingredient in the pursuit of holistic well-being and beauty.

Neem in Industrial Applications: Harnessing Nature's Versatility

Beyond its traditional and agricultural uses, neem (*Azadirachta indica*) finds a place in various industrial applications, showcasing its versatility and eco-friendly attributes. Here's an exploration of neem's role in industrial settings:

Biopesticides and Insecticides:

Agricultural Sector: Neem-derived biopesticides and insecticides are widely utilized in agriculture. They offer an effective and sustainable alternative to synthetic chemicals, contributing to integrated pest management practices.

Soap and Detergent Production:

Saponins in Neem: Neem contains natural surfactants called saponins. Extracts rich in saponins are used in soap and detergent manufacturing, enhancing their cleansing properties.

Cosmetic and Personal Care Ingredients:

Skincare and Haircare Products: Neem oil and extracts are incorporated into cosmetic formulations such as lotions, creams, shampoos, and conditioners. Their antimicrobial and nourishing properties contribute to these products.

Pharmaceutical Industry:

Medicinal Extracts: Neem's medicinal compounds are harnessed for pharmaceutical purposes. Azadirachtin, nimbin, and nimbidin are studied for their potential in developing medications for various health conditions.

Neem Coatings for Wood and Metal:

Anti-Termite Treatment: Neem oil is used as a natural coating for wood, providing protection against termites and other pests. It serves as an eco-friendly alternative to chemical wood preservatives.

Corrosion Resistance: Neem-based coatings are explored for their potential in protecting metal surfaces from corrosion.

Adhesive and Gum Production:

Tannins in Neem Bark: Neem bark, rich in tannins, is used in the production of adhesives and gums. Tannins contribute to the adhesive properties and durability of these products.

Neem Biofuel:

Biodiesel Production: Neem oil has been explored as a potential feedstock for biodiesel production. Its high fatty acid content makes it a viable candidate for sustainable biofuel.

Water Purification:

Natural Flocculant: Neem seeds contain proteins that act as natural flocculants. Crushed neem seeds have been used as a traditional method to clarify water by settling impurities.

Neem-Based Inks and Dyes:

Eco-Friendly Printing: Neem extracts are used in the formulation of eco-friendly inks. The natural pigments present in neem contribute to the coloration of textiles and paper.

Neem-Based Fertilizers:

Organic Agriculture: Neem cake, a by-product of neem oil extraction, serves as an organic fertilizer. It enriches the soil with nutrients and supports sustainable farming practices.

Leather Industry:

Tannin Extraction: Neem bark, rich in tannins, is utilized in the leather industry for tanning hides. Tannins contribute to the preservation and quality of leather.

Neem's integration into various industrial processes reflects its adaptability and eco-friendly nature. As industries increasingly prioritize sustainable practices, neem emerges as a valuable resource, offering effective solutions that align with environmental and social responsibility.

CHAPTER 7
NEEM IN TRADITIONAL AND MODERN MEDICINE

Neem in Folk Remedies: Time-Honored Wisdom for Well-Being

Neem (*Azadirachta indica*) has a rich history steeped in traditional medicine, where it has been revered as a versatile healer in numerous cultures. Folk remedies centered around neem draw upon its various parts, from leaves and bark to seeds and oil, to address a spectrum of health concerns. Here's an exploration of neem's role in folk remedies:

Skin Conditions:

Acne and Pimples: Neem leaves and neem oil are often used in folk remedies to create pastes or tonics for managing acne. The antimicrobial properties of neem help combat bacteria associated with skin blemishes.

Eczema and Psoriasis: Neem-based ointments or creams are applied to alleviate symptoms of eczema and psoriasis. The anti-inflammatory compounds in neem contribute to soothing irritated skin.

Oral Health:

Gum Infections and Cavities: Chewing neem twigs has been a traditional practice for maintaining oral hygiene. Neem's antibacterial properties are believed to combat gum infections and help prevent cavities.

Mouth Ulcers: Rinsing the mouth with neem-infused water is a folk remedy for managing mouth ulcers, leveraging neem's antimicrobial effects.

Fever and Malaria:

Fever Reduction: Neem leaves are used in decoctions or infusions for their antipyretic properties, offering a folk remedy for reducing fever.

Antimalarial Use: Traditional practices involve using neem-based preparations for their potential antimalarial effects, contributing to malaria management.

Digestive Health:

Parasitic Infections: Neem is employed in folk remedies to address gastrointestinal issues caused by parasites. Neem extracts are believed to have a cleansing effect on the digestive tract.

Indigestion and Bloating: Neem-based formulations are sometimes used to alleviate indigestion and bloating, tapping into neem's digestive benefits.

Immune Support:

Immune-Boosting Tonics: Neem is incorporated into folk remedies to prepare tonics believed to support the immune system. These tonics may be consumed during periods of illness or as preventive measures.

Joint Pain and Arthritis:

Anti-Inflammatory Pastes: Neem oil or neem leaf pastes are used topically in folk remedies to alleviate joint pain and symptoms associated with arthritis. Nimbin and other compounds in neem contribute to its anti-inflammatory effects.

Hair and Scalp Conditions:

Dandruff and Scalp Irritation: Neem oil is applied to the scalp in folk remedies to address dandruff and soothe scalp irritation. Its antifungal properties contribute to a healthier scalp.

Hair Growth Stimulant: Some traditional practices involve using neem-infused oils or pastes to stimulate hair growth and maintain overall hair health.

Wound Healing:

Antibacterial Balms: Neem-based ointments or balms are applied to wounds and cuts in folk remedies for their potential antibacterial properties.

Neem's ability to support wound healing is attributed to compounds like nimbidin.

Folk remedies involving neem reflect a profound understanding of its medicinal properties passed down through generations. While modern research continues to explore and validate these traditional uses, neem remains a revered botanical ally in the realm of natural and holistic well-being.

Scientific Research and Discoveries on Neem (*Azadirachta indica*): Unlocking Nature's Secrets

The scientific exploration of neem has uncovered a wealth of knowledge about its bioactive compounds and potential applications across various fields. Researchers have delved into the intricate chemistry of neem and unveiled its therapeutic, agricultural, and industrial potential. Here's a glimpse into the scientific research and discoveries surrounding neem:

Antimicrobial Properties:

Key Compound Azadirachtin: Scientific studies have confirmed the potent antimicrobial effects of azadirachtin, a major compound in neem. Neem extracts have demonstrated efficacy against bacteria, viruses, and fungi, inspiring the development of natural antimicrobial agents.

Agricultural Applications:

Biopesticides and Insecticidal Properties: Neem's role in pest control has been extensively studied. Azadirachtin disrupts insect feeding and molting, making neem a valuable component in biopesticides. This research supports sustainable agriculture practices, reducing reliance on synthetic pesticides.

Medicinal Properties:

Antidiabetic Potential: Scientific investigations have explored neem's potential in managing diabetes. Compounds like nimbidin and quercetin are studied for their role in regulating blood sugar levels, paving the way for potential therapeutic applications.

Immunomodulatory Effects:

Polysaccharides and Immune Support: Studies have identified polysaccharides in neem with immunomodulatory effects. These findings contribute to understanding neem's traditional use for immune support and may have implications in immune-related therapies.

Anticancer Research:

Triterpenoids in Cancer Treatment: Triterpenoids found in neem, including gedunin and azadiradione, have been subjects of research for their potential anticancer properties. Studies suggest that neem compounds may inhibit the growth of cancer cells and induce apoptosis.

Skin Health and Dermatology:

Anti-Inflammatory and Antioxidant Effects: Scientific studies have validated neem's anti-inflammatory and antioxidant properties, supporting its traditional use in skincare. Neem's potential in managing skin conditions such as acne, eczema, and psoriasis is a focus of ongoing research.

Environmental Impact:

Neem-Based Pesticides and Ecological Balance: Research has explored the environmental impact of neem-based pesticides. Their low toxicity to non-target organisms and biodegradability contribute to ecological balance, aligning with sustainable agricultural practices.

Neem in Dental Care:

Antibacterial Effects in Oral Health: Scientific studies have investigated neem's antibacterial effects in dental care. Neem-based oral care products, including toothpaste and mouthwash, show promise in promoting oral hygiene.

Antiviral Potential:

Triterpenoids and Antiviral Effects: Some neem triterpenoids have demonstrated antiviral potential in scientific studies. Research explores the use of neem compounds in developing antiviral therapies.

Biodiesel Production:

Feasibility as Biodiesel Feedstock: Research has assessed the feasibility of using neem oil as a feedstock for biodiesel production. Its high fatty acid content makes it a potential candidate for sustainable biofuel.

Scientific research on neem continues to expand, providing a foundation for its integration into modern medicine, agriculture, and industry. The discoveries underscore neem's potential as a sustainable and multifaceted resource with implications for human health, environmental stewardship, and economic development.

CHAPTER 8
SUSTAINABLE FARMING WITH NEEM

Neem in Organic Agriculture: A Green Revolution in Sustainable Farming

Neem (*Azadirachta indica*) stands as a cornerstone in the realm of organic agriculture, offering a natural arsenal that promotes sustainable farming practices. Its multifaceted benefits, ranging from pest control to soil enrichment, have positioned neem as a green ally for farmers committed to ecological balance. Here's an exploration of neem's pivotal role in organic agriculture:

Biopesticidal Marvel:

Azadirachtin Powerhouse: Neem's biopesticidal properties, primarily attributed to azadirachtin, serve as a cornerstone in organic pest management. Azadirachtin disrupts the feeding and reproductive patterns of insects, providing an effective and eco-friendly alternative to synthetic pesticides.

Non-Toxic to Beneficial Organisms:

Preserving Natural Predators: Neem-based pesticides are selective in their action, posing minimal harm to beneficial insects, pollinators, and other non-target organisms. This specificity supports the preservation of ecological balance within agricultural ecosystems.

Nematode Control:

Nimbin's Nematode Resistance: Neem's nematode-controlling properties, particularly attributed to compounds like nimbin, contribute to soil health in organic agriculture. By managing nematode populations, neem supports the well-being of crops and enhances overall yield.

Fungal Disease Management:

Antifungal Arsenal: Neem's antifungal compounds, including azadirachtin, help prevent and manage fungal diseases in crops. Organic farmers rely on neem-based formulations to combat issues such as powdery mildew and rust.

Soil Enrichment with Neem Cake:

Organic Fertilizer Supplement: Neem cake, a by-product of neem oil extraction, serves as a valuable organic fertilizer. Rich in nutrients, neem cake enhances soil fertility, improves microbial activity, and promotes sustainable agricultural practices.

Integrated Pest Management (IPM):

Balanced Approach: Neem fits seamlessly into the principles of Integrated Pest Management (IPM) in organic agriculture. By combining cultural, biological, and mechanical controls with neem-based pesticides, farmers adopt a holistic and sustainable approach to pest management.

Resistance Management:

Combating Pesticide Resistance: Neem's complex composition makes it challenging for pests to develop resistance, unlike conventional pesticides. This attribute supports long-term efficacy in organic farming and reduces the risk of resistance development.

Agroforestry and Biodiversity:

Neem Trees in Agroforestry: Integrating neem trees into agroforestry systems contributes to biodiversity. Neem's presence provides shade, windbreaks, and additional organic matter, fostering a more resilient and diverse agricultural landscape.

Sustainable Practices in Neem Oil Extraction:

Reduced Environmental Impact: Organic agriculture extends to the methods used in neem oil extraction. Adopting sustainable practices minimizes the environmental impact, ensuring that the entire process aligns with organic farming principles.

Consumer Confidence and Residue-Free Produce:

Meeting Organic Standards: Neem's natural origins and low environmental impact resonate with consumers seeking organic produce. The use of neem in organic agriculture aligns with the demand for residue-free, sustainable farming practices.

Neem's integration into organic agriculture epitomizes a harmonious relationship between nature and farming. As organic practices gain prominence, neem emerges as a key player in fostering sustainable, environmentally conscious, and resilient agricultural systems around the world.

Agroforestry Practices: Cultivating Harmony Between Agriculture and Forestry

Agroforestry is a sustainable land-use system that integrates trees and shrubs into agricultural landscapes, fostering a harmonious coexistence between traditional farming practices and forestry. This innovative approach offers a myriad of benefits, combining the productivity of agriculture with the ecological diversity and resilience provided by trees. Here's an exploration of key agroforestry practices:

Alley Cropping:

Integration of Crops and Trees: Alley cropping involves planting rows of trees with crop plants in the alleys between them. This system provides shade, windbreaks, and organic matter from tree litter, enhancing soil fertility and crop yields.

Silvopasture:

Integrating Livestock and Trees: Silvopasture combines trees, forage, and livestock in a symbiotic system. Trees provide shade for animals, forage quality improves in the presence of trees, and the integration enhances carbon sequestration.

Windbreaks and Shelterbelts:

Protecting Crops from Wind: Planting rows of trees as windbreaks or shelterbelts shields crops from strong winds, reducing soil erosion and creating a microclimate that benefits crop growth.

Forest Garden Systems:

Biodiversity-Rich Agriculture: Forest garden systems mimic natural forests, incorporating a variety of fruit trees, shrubs, and crops. This diverse mix promotes ecological balance, pest control, and resilience to climatic variations.

Agroforestry for Soil Conservation:

Preventing Soil Erosion: Trees with deep root systems help bind soil particles, preventing erosion. This is particularly beneficial on sloping lands where erosion is a concern.

Taungya System:

Sequential Land Use: The Taungya system involves planting crops alongside young trees. As the trees grow, the crop area is gradually reduced. This sequential approach maximizes land use efficiency while promoting reforestation.

Agroforestry for Water Management:

Riparian Buffer Zones: Planting trees along water bodies creates riparian buffer zones. These zones filter runoff, reduce nutrient loading, and enhance water quality.

Homegardens:

Diverse Mini-Farms: Homegardens integrate trees, shrubs, and crops around homesteads. This system provides a year-round supply of diverse foods, supporting food security and enhancing household resilience.

Agroforestry and Carbon Sequestration:

Contributing to Climate Mitigation: Trees in agroforestry systems act as carbon sinks, sequestering carbon dioxide from the atmosphere. This makes agroforestry an ally in climate change mitigation efforts.

Multi-Strata Agroforestry:

Vertical Layers of Vegetation: Multi-strata agroforestry involves planting different layers of vegetation, from tall trees to ground cover crops. This maximizes resource use efficiency, light capture, and biodiversity.

Timber and Non-Timber Forest Products:

Balancing Production and Conservation: Agroforestry systems that include timber and non-timber forest products provide economic benefits while maintaining forest cover and biodiversity.

Agroforestry practices exemplify a holistic approach to land management, blending the best aspects of agriculture and forestry. As the world seeks sustainable and resilient solutions to food production and environmental conservation, agroforestry emerges as a model that not only meets these challenges but also enriches the landscapes it touches.

CHAPTER 9

CHALLENGES AND FUTURE PROSPECTS

Environmental Concerns: Navigating Challenges for a Sustainable Future

The world faces a myriad of environmental concerns, reflecting the complex interactions between human activities and the delicate balance of Earth's ecosystems. Addressing these issues is crucial for building a sustainable future. Here's an overview of some prominent environmental concerns:

Climate Change:

Rising Temperatures: Human-induced activities, primarily the burning of fossil fuels, deforestation, and industrial processes, contribute to the buildup of greenhouse gases in the atmosphere. This leads to global warming, altering climate patterns, and causing extreme weather events.

Loss of Biodiversity:

Habitat Destruction: Deforestation, urbanization, and intensive agriculture disrupt natural habitats, leading to a loss of biodiversity. Species extinction rates are accelerating, posing risks to ecosystems and diminishing the resilience of natural systems.

Deforestation:

Ecosystem Disruption: Clearing forests for agriculture, logging, and infrastructure development has far-reaching consequences. Deforestation not only contributes to habitat loss but also reduces carbon sequestration capacity, exacerbating climate change.

Pollution:

Air, Water, and Soil Contamination: Industrial emissions, improper waste disposal, and excessive use of chemical fertilizers and pesticides contribute to air, water, and soil pollution. This poses risks to human health, ecosystems, and wildlife.

Overexploitation of Natural Resources:

Depleting Finite Resources: Unsustainable extraction of resources such as freshwater, minerals, and fisheries can lead to their depletion. Overexploitation disrupts ecosystems and jeopardizes the livelihoods of communities dependent on these resources.

Plastic Pollution:

Persistent Environmental Threat: Improper disposal and excessive use of plastic contribute to widespread pollution in oceans and terrestrial environments. Microplastics, posing threats to marine life and ecosystems, are a growing concern.

Land Degradation:

Loss of Arable Land: Unsustainable agricultural practices, deforestation, and urbanization contribute to land degradation. Soil erosion, desertification, and loss of arable land compromise food security and ecosystem health.

Ocean Acidification:

Carbon Dioxide Absorption: Excess carbon dioxide in the atmosphere is absorbed by the oceans, leading to increased acidity. Ocean acidification poses risks to marine life, particularly organisms with calcium carbonate shells and skeletons.

Resource Scarcity:

Growing Demand: Increasing global populations and resource-intensive lifestyles contribute to resource scarcity. This includes water scarcity, depletion of fisheries, and strain on essential resources needed for human well-being.

Air Quality Decline:

Urbanization and Industrial Emissions: Rapid urbanization and industrial activities contribute to poor air quality. Air pollution, including particulate matter and pollutants like nitrogen oxides, has adverse effects on human health and ecosystems.

Addressing these environmental concerns requires concerted efforts at local, national, and global levels. Sustainable practices, conservation initiatives, and policy measures are essential to mitigate the impact of human activities on the environment and pave the way for a more balanced and resilient planet.

Innovations and Research Directions: Paving the Way for a Sustainable Tomorrow

As humanity confronts pressing environmental challenges, innovations and research directions play a pivotal role in shaping a sustainable future. From renewable energy solutions to cutting-edge conservation technologies, ongoing efforts are geared towards fostering resilience and minimizing our ecological footprint. Here's a glimpse into some key innovations and research directions:

Renewable Energy Advancements:

Solar Power Breakthroughs: Ongoing research focuses on enhancing the efficiency and affordability of solar energy. Innovations include next-gen solar cells, advanced photovoltaic technologies, and energy storage solutions, contributing to a transition towards cleaner energy sources.

Circular Economy Models:

Waste-to-Resource Strategies: Innovations in circular economy models aim to minimize waste and maximize resource efficiency. From recycling technologies to closed-loop systems, these approaches address resource scarcity and reduce environmental impact.

Sustainable Agriculture Technologies:

Precision Farming: Advances in precision farming technologies, including AI-driven systems and IoT applications, optimize resource use in agriculture. This enhances crop yields, reduces environmental impact, and promotes sustainable farming practices.

Green Transportation Solutions:

Electrification and Sustainable Mobility: Research in electric vehicles, alternative fuels, and smart transportation systems aims to reduce the carbon footprint of the transportation sector. Innovations include battery technologies, charging infrastructure, and efficient public transport systems.

Conservation Drones and Remote Sensing:

Monitoring Ecosystems: Conservation efforts benefit from innovations in drones and remote sensing technologies. These tools enable real-time monitoring of ecosystems, helping researchers and conservationists make informed decisions for biodiversity conservation.

Sustainable Urban Planning:

Smart Cities: Research in sustainable urban planning focuses on creating smart cities that prioritize energy efficiency, green spaces, and smart infrastructure. These innovations aim to enhance urban resilience and reduce the environmental impact of urbanization.

Biotechnology for Environmental Cleanup:

Bioremediation: Biotechnological innovations, such as genetically modified microorganisms, offer promising solutions for environmental cleanup. These approaches target pollutants and contaminants, contributing to soil and water remediation.

Climate-Resilient Crop Varieties:

Climate-Smart Agriculture: Research on developing climate-resilient crop varieties helps farmers adapt to changing climatic conditions. This includes crops that are drought-resistant, heat-tolerant, and adapted to varying environmental stressors.

Ocean Conservation Technologies:

Autonomous Underwater Vehicles (AUVs): AUVs are revolutionizing ocean exploration and conservation. These autonomous vehicles assist in mapping the ocean floor, studying marine biodiversity, and monitoring the impacts of climate change on marine ecosystems.

Carbon Capture and Storage (CCS):

Mitigating Greenhouse Gas Emissions: CCS technologies aim to capture carbon dioxide emissions from industrial processes and power plants. Ongoing research explores efficient methods for capturing, transporting, and safely storing CO2 to mitigate climate change.

Nature-Based Solutions:

Ecosystem Restoration: Nature-based solutions involve restoring and protecting ecosystems to address environmental challenges. This includes reforestation initiatives, wetland restoration, and the creation of green infrastructure for sustainable urban development.

Eco-Friendly Materials:

Biodegradable Plastics: Innovations in eco-friendly materials focus on developing biodegradable alternatives to traditional plastics. These materials aim to reduce the environmental impact of plastic pollution.

These innovations and research directions underscore the commitment to finding sustainable solutions to complex environmental challenges. By harnessing the power of technology, science, and creative thinking, researchers and innovators contribute to building a resilient and environmentally conscious future for generations to come.